Published By Nicholas Thompson

@ Tony Davis

Wheat Belly Diet: The Ultimate Guide to Losing

Weight and Feeling Energized

ISBN 978-1-990666-93-3

I0558143

TABLE OF CONTENTS

Ginger & Chilli Curry 1

Thai Coconut Stew 3

Stuffed Peppers 5

Turkey Club Sandwich 7

Delicious Fish Sticks 8

Beef Meat Loaf 10

Zucchini Rice 13

Cucumber Sandwich Bites 16

Berry Coconut Smoothie 17

Spiced Berry & Citrus Oatmeal 18

Citrus Salmon Fillets With Onion 20

Snicker Doodles 23

Walnut Cherry Almond Flour Cookies 25

Apple Cranberry Stuffed Pork Roast 27

Apricot Chicken 29

Potato Salad With Peas And Green Beans 31

Asparagus And Avocado Salad 33

Creamy Cauliflower Salad 34

Crepes With Ricotta And Strawberries........................... 35

Basic Pie Crust 38

Meatballs With Tomato Sauce 41

Ham And Egg Breakfast Meal... 44

Delicious Shrimp Bisque 46

Chicken And Wild Rice Soup... 48

Chicken And Dumplings.. 50

Homemade Granola Bar.. 53

Trail Mix Snacks 55

Spicy Party Mix Wheat Free Snacks 56

Onion, Garlic & Kale 58

Quinoa & Black Beans 60

Chocolate Dipped Walnut And Currant Cookies 62

Gingerbread People 65

Asparagus Frittata 67

Baby Bok Choy With Cashews 69

Baked Beans In Tomato Sauce 70

Vegetable Stir-Fry 72

Chicken With Prunes And Green Olives 74

Mushroom Frittata With Broccoli 77

Mushroom Frittata With Artichokes 80

Parmesan Cheese Soufflé 83

Onion Rings 86

Eggplant-Veggie Snacks 88

Delicious Fish Sticks 90

Tasty Creamy Parmesan Chicken 92

Glazed Pork Tenderloin 94

Beaded Pork Chops 96

Glazed Salmon 98

Vegetable Chili 99

Toffee Almond Flour Cookies 102

Peanut Butter Almond Flour Cookies 104

Chicken Marbella 106

Chipotle Lime Bacon-Wrapped Shrimp 108

Banana-Raspberry With Coconut Milk And Sunflower
Seeds 110

Quinoa-Orange Porridge 111

Mixed Berries With Yogurt And Pumpkin Seeds 112

Green Chile Strata 114

Green Pepper Omelet With Spinach 117

Sausage Bits Snack 120

Chickpeas Snack 122

Coco-Nutty, Limey, Grilled Pineapples 124

Sweet Peach Crisp 125

Sweet Macaroons 127

Pineapple Tapioca 129

Cheese Fondue 131

Garlic & Bay Tilapia 133

Strawberry & Banana Smoothie 135

Shrimp Cake 136

Cod Picasa 138

Chicken Parmesan 140

Ginger & Chilli Curry

Ingredients:

- 3 garlic cloves

- 1 ½ inch root ginger

- 1 red chilli

- A pinch of salt

- 500g frozen spinach

- 2 tablespoons vegetable oil

- 2 plantain

- 2 small onions

- Fresh coriander

Directions:

1. Peel and slice the plantain and onions.

2. Crush the garlic cloves and peel and grate the ginger. Chop the chili finely.
3. In a large skillet, heat the vegetable oil for a moment.
4. Fry the plantain and onion for 5 minutes, or until soft and golden. Add the garlic, ginger, chili and a pinch of salt. Fry for another 2-3 minutes.
5. Next, combine the spinach with the skillet contents and half a cup of water.
6. Cook for 25 minutes, stirring every 5 or so minutes.
7. Serve with pita bread.

Thai Coconut Stew

Ingredients:

- 1 mild jalapeno

- 400ml coconut milk

- 2 garlic cloves

- 1 cube of vegetable stock

- 1 teaspoon cayenne pepper

- 1 large sweet potato

- 500g kidney beans

- Lime juice

- A pinch of salt

- Fresh cilantro

Directions:

1. Peel and chop the sweet potato into bite size chunks.

2. In a large skillet combine all the Ingredients:, with exception to the cilantro.

3. Bring to the boil and then simmer over low heat for 30 minutes or until the potatoes are soft throughout.

4. Mash the potatoes into the rest of the stew and serve with fresh cilantro.

5. Serve with vegan friendly bread.

Stuffed Peppers

Ingredients:

- ½ cup onion, slashed

- 1 cup cilantro, slashed

- 1 tsp. stew powder

- 2 tsp. cumin

- 8 sweet chime peppers

- 500 g. turkey, ground

- 100 g. green chillies, diced

- Salt

Directions:

1. Blend all the fixings in a medium dish, with the exception of the sweet chime peppers.
2. Cut off the highest point of the ringer peppers and put aside.

3. Stuff the bigger 50% of the peppers with the turkey mixture.
4. Place the stuffed ringer peppers in a preparing dish and spread with the tops that was situated aside.
5. Heat for 60 minutes at a 350 degree temperature. Serve while hot.

Turkey Club Sandwich

Ingredients:

- 1 cluster romaine lettuce

- 1 avocado, cut

- Dijon mustard 500 g.

- 2 cuts basic bread as explained
  earlier

- Turkey breast, broiled

Directions:

1. Toast the basic bread cuts. On one bread cut,
   spread on the Dijon mustard.
2. Place two or more cuts of avocados. Put on
   the lettuce, then two or three cuts of the
   simmered turkey.
3. Spread with the other bread cut. Serve with
   your favourite sauce.

Delicious Fish Sticks

Ingredients:

- 6 tbsp. Olive oil

- 1 cup almond flour

- 1/2 kg. White fish fillet

- 2 eggs

- Salt

Directions:

1. Flush the cuts of fish and place on a plate. Uproot the bones of the fish and cut into 1 by 5 inch rectangles.
2. Blend the flour and salt in one bowl, the eggs in a different dish.
3. Dunk the fish into the eggs in the first place, then into the flour rapidly.
4. Set up all the fish in this way on a plate.

5. Over medium warmth, warm a pan with three tablespoons of olive oil.

6. Place 50% of the fish fillets on the pan sufficiently leaving space to turn them over and cook.

7. Cook every side of the fish until chestnut. Serve with your favourite sauce or ketchup.

Beef Meat Loaf

Ingredients:

- 2 cloves garlic, minced

- 2 pounds ground beef

- ¼ cup ground flaxseeds

- 2 extensive eggs

- ½ cup tomato juice

- 2 tablespoons hacked parsley

- 1 teaspoon ocean salt

- 2 tablespoons olive or coconut oil

- 1 little onion, finely cleaved

- 1 carrot, finely cleaved

- 1 rib celery, finely cleaved

- ½ teaspoon ground black pepper

- 4 strips bacon, cut down the middle

Directions:

1. Preheat the oven to 350°F.

2. Daintily oil a rimmed baking sheet. In an extensive skillet over medium warmth, warm the oil.

3. Cook the onion, carrot, celery, and garlic, mixing infrequently, for 5 minutes, or until delicate.

4. Exchange to an expansive bowl and let cool to room temperature. Include the beef, flaxseeds, eggs, tomato juice, parsley, salt, and pepper to the dish. Mix completely.

5. Exchange the mixture to the baking sheet and shape into a log around 9" × 5" using your hands. Lay the bacon strips the long way over the top and sides.

6. Press to follow. Heat for 1 hour 15 minutes, or until a thermometer embedded in the middle registers 160° F and the meat is no more pink in colour. Let rest for 10 minutes prior to cutting into slices.

Zucchini Rice

Ingredients:

- 1 teaspoon of butter

- 1/2 teaspoon cumin seeds

- 1/2 teaspoon black mustard seeds

- 4 red peppers entirety

- 2 Bay leaves

- 1/2 teaspoon of salt

- Little piece of cinnamon stick around 1/2 inch

- 1 cup rice

- 2 cups water

- 1 cup destroyed zucchini with skin

- 1 tablespoon of oil

- 1 teaspoon of lemon juice

Directions:

1. Heat the oil and butter in an overwhelming saucepan over medium high warmth.

2. Test the warmth by adding one cumin seed to oil; if the cumin breaks immediately oil is prepared.

3. Include cumin seeds and mustard seeds to the oil.

4. After seeds break include red pepper and bay while it clears out. Include rice and panfry for around 2 minutes.

5. Include water, zucchini, salt and lemon juice. Mix and convey to boil.

6. After rice reaches boiling point turn the warmth down to low and spread the pan.

7. Cook rice for around 15 minutes or until the rice is delicate and the water has dissipated.

8. Serve as may be, with soup, yogurt, and pickle.

9. Spread some cheddar cheese over the rice before serving.

Cucumber Sandwich Bites

Ingredients:

- 4 pcs. deli turkey sclies

- 4 slices of cheese singles

- 1 pc. cucumber

Directions:

1. Remove the skin of the cucumber and cut into slices.
2. Cut the turkey slices and cheese into bite size pieces
3. Lay the slices of cucumber and top with turkey slice and cheese.
4. Sandwich with another slice of cucumber. Enjoy snacking.

Berry Coconut Smoothie

Ingredients:

- 1 tbsp. unsweetened dark cocoa powder

- 1 tbsp. cinnamon powder

- 1 cup ice

- ½ cup banana peeled

- ½ cup blueberry

- ½ avocado pitted, chopped

- 1/3 cup coconut milk

Directions:

1. Blend all the Ingredients: in a blender until smooth. Enjoy immediately.

Spiced Berry & Citrus Oatmeal

Ingredients:

- ¼ tsp ground turmeric

- A pinch of ginger

- ½ tsp cinnamon

- ½ cup frozen blueberries

- 1 cup water

- ¼ cup orange juice

- 3/4 cup oats

- ¼ cup dried cranberries

Directions:

1. Mix together the cranberries, blueberries oats and cinnamon, turmeric and ginger in a heat-proof bowl.

2. Toss in the water and stir once more to incorporate.

3. Cook on a high temperature for 1 minute. Remove and stir briefly.

4. Cook for another minute and remove. Stir once more.

5. Add the orange juice gradually, ensuring you do not make the consistency too thin.

6. Heat for 15-20 seconds more and serve immediately.

Citrus Salmon Fillets With Onion

Ingredients:

- 2 tsp lemon pepper

- 2 tsp garlic powder

- 2 oranges, sliced

- 1 onion, thinly sliced

- 1 tbsp dried parsley

- ½ cup orange juice

- 4 tsp lemon juice

- 1 ½ tbsp olive oil

- 5 salmon fillets

- 1 tbsp dried parsley

- ½ cup orange juice

- 1 tbsp hone

Directions:

1. Preheat the oven to 400F.
2. Combine lemon pepper, parsley and garlic powder in a mixing bowl.
3. In a 9*13 baking dish, arrange the sliced orange into a layer.
4. On the top of the orange layer arrange the sliced onion in a similar manner.
5. Dress with the olive oil and roughly half of the parsley mixture prepared earlier.
6. Put the baking dish in the oven and cook for 25 minutes, or until the onions have browned.
7. Set aside the tray for later and raise the oven temperature to 450F.
8. Gently man oeuvre the onion and orange in the try aside, making a well in the middle of the tray.
9. Rest the salmon fillets in the well. Garnish with the rest of the parsley mixture.

10. In a mixing bowl, combine the orange juice, lemon juice and honey. Use this mixture to coat the salmon.

11. Roast for 15 minutes in the oven.

12. Separate the orange from the onion. Serve the salmon and onion mixture.

Snicker Doodles

Ingredients:

- 1/3 cup melted palm shortening

- 1 ½ tbsp vanilla extract

- 2 cups fine ground almond flour

- ¼ tsp baking soda

- ¼ cup mild honey

For the cinnamon coating:

- 2 tbsp ground cinnamon

- 2 tbsp raw coconut crystals

Directions:

1. Preheat the oven to 350 degrees.
2. Place parchment paper on the baking sheet.
3. Combine and stir the dry ingredients together in a medium bowl.

4. In a separate bowl, combine the vanilla, oil and honey.
5. Add the wet ingredients to the flour mixture and stir to combine. Allow to rest for few minutes until it thickens.
6. Combine the sugar crystals and ground cinnamon in a bowl.
7. Use clean hands or a rounded spoon to scoop dough. Gently form it into a ball and roll it in your palms. Sprinkle with the cinnamon mixture.
8. Place the balls into the baking sheet lined with parchment paper.
9. Space each ball about 3 inches apart.
10. Flatten the cookie with your hand.
11. Bake in the oven for 8 minutes at 350 degrees.
12. Leave the cookies on the baking sheet and allow to cool.

Walnut Cherry Almond Flour Cookies

Ingredients:

- 2/3 cup dried cherries

- 1/3 cup dark chocolate chips

- ½ cup sugar

- ½ tsp salt

- 1 tsp vanilla

- 2/3 cup chopped walnuts

- 3 cups almond flour

- ½ cup butter

- 1/3 cup applesauce

- ½ tsp baking powder

Directions:

1. Preheat the oven to 350 degrees.

2. Mix the almond flour, applesauce, butter, salt, vanilla, baking powder and sugar in a food processor and blend until it is smooth.
3. Add the cherries, chocolate chips and walnuts.
4. Scoop the dough into your palm and form into balls.
5. Bake the balls for 15 minutes. Remember to watch it closely because it tends to brown quickly.
6. Place on the rack to cool.

Apple Cranberry Stuffed Pork Roast

Ingredients:

Filling

- ½ cup cranberries

- 1 tbsp grated ginger

- 1 tbsp yellow mustard seed

- 1/8 cayenne pepper

- ½ tsp ground all spice

- 1 cup apple cider

- ¾ cup brown sugar

- ½ cup cider vinegar

- 1 large thinly sliced shallot

- 1 ½ cup dried apples

Pork roast

- 2 ½ boneless pork loin

- Salt and pepper to taste

Directions:

1. Combine all filling ingredients in a pan over medium heat.

2. Cook until apples are soft. Strain and reserve the liquid.

3. Return the liquid into the saucepan and simmer for about 5 minutes. Set aside.

4. Cut the pork in a double butterfly style and season with salt and pepper.

5. Spread the filling on top of the roast and roll it up tightly and tie with a twine.

6. Roast the meat in the oven for 45 to 60 minutes in 130 degrees.

7. Brush the meat with the liquid reserved from boiling the filling and cook for 5 more minutes. Slice into pieces then serve.

Apricot Chicken

Ingredients:

- 2 cups chicken stock

- 1 chopped onion

- 1 tbsp chopped rosemary

- 1 tsp cinnamon

- 2 tsp hot sauce

- Salt and pepper to taste

- 1 ½ lb chopped apricots

- ¼ cup sugar

- 2 tbsp cider vinegar

- 2 lb skinless chicken

- 1 tbsp unsalted butter

- 3 tbsp olive oil

Directions:

1. Mix chopped apricots, sugar and vinegar in a bowl and marinate.
2. In a large pan, heat the olive oil and butter. Cook the chicken then set aside.
3. Add the remaining oil and sauté the onion until it wilts. Gently add the chicken stock then simmer.
4. Puree 2/3 of the apricots along with its juices. Pour the puree in the pan then add the stock and onions.
5. Add in cinnamon, Tabasco, rosemary and salt. Simmer for 20 minutes.
6. Put the chicken and apricot pieces then simmer for 5 minutes.

Potato Salad With Peas And Green Beans

Ingredients:

- 100g garden peas, fresh or frozen

- 100g watercress, washed

- 50g pea shoots (or baby spinach)

- 1 bunch radish, sliced in fine strips

- 1 tsp of fresh lemon juice, preferably extracted from ½ large-sized lemon

- 2 tbsp flax oil

- 5-8 pcs mint leaves, finely chopped

- 500g baby new potatoes (or marble potatoes), sliced into halves

- 200g green beans, topped and tailed

- Water

- Salt and pepper to season

Directions:

1. Put the halved potatoes in a saucepan with cold water, and bring to a boil.
2. Let simmer for 10 minutes, or until potatoes are tender.
3. Drain and place potatoes in a serving bowl, and season with salt and ground black pepper.
4. Boil another 2-3 cups of water to a boil, add the beans and let simmer for 90 seconds.
5. Add the peas, and let simmer for another 90 seconds. Drain and add to the potatoes.
6. Add the watercress, pea shoots (or spinach), and radishes.
7. In a separate bowl, whisk the lemon juice, flax oil and finely chopped mint.
8. Season with black pepper. Pour the mixture over the salad.
9. Toss and serve. This makes 2-3 servings.

Asparagus And Avocado Salad

Ingredients:

- 1 pc cucumber, sliced

- ½ pc avocado, sliced

- 2 sprigs of asparagus

- 2 bunches or handfuls of mixed salad greens, fresh or frozen, sliced

- 1 pc tomato, sliced

Directions:

1. In a bowl, place salad greens, tomato and cucumber. Mix lightly.
2. Top with avocado and asparagus. Toss, then serve.

Creamy Cauliflower Salad

Ingredients:

- 5 tbsp mayonnaise, low-fat option

- 2 tbsp cider vinegar

- 1 pc shallot, finely chopped

- ¼ tsp ground pepper

- 3 cups cauliflower florets, chopped

- 2 cups romaine, heart part, chopped

- 1 pc red apple, chopped

Directions:

1. In a large bowl, whisk mayonnaise, vinegar, shallot, and ground pepper, until smooth.
2. Add in cauliflower florets, romaine, and apple slices. Toss. This makes 5-6 servings.

Crepes With Ricotta And Strawberries

Ingredients:

Filling

- 1 cup ricotta

- 1 teaspoon xylitol or 1 drop liquid stevia or to desired sweetness

- 1 teaspoon lemon peel

- 2 cups strawberries, halved

Crepes

- ¼ cup coconut flour

- ¼ cup golden flaxseed meal

- ¼ teaspoon sea salt

- 1½ cups almond or carton-variety coconut milk

- 4 eggs

- ¼ teaspoon vanilla extract

Directions:

To prepare the filling:

1. In a small bowl, mix the ricotta, Xylitol or stevia, and lemon peel and then set aside for later use.

To cook the crepes:

2. In a large bowl, mix the coconut flour, flaxseed meal, and salt. In a modest bowl, whisk together the milk, eggs, and vanilla.

3. Now, add the egg mixture to the flour mixture and stir until combined.

4. Coat a small non-stick frying pan with oil and heat over medium high temperature.

5. Measure ⅓ cup of the Batter and pour into the pan, swirling the batter around so it coats the underside of the pan.

6. Cook for 3 minutes, or until the tip of the crepe looks dry.
7. Move around the crepe and cook for 1 min, or until the bottom is dry.
8. Repetition with the remaining batter, stacking the Crepes as they are prepared.
9. Top each crepe with 2 tablespoons of the ricotta filling and ¼ cup of the strawberries.

Basic Pie Crust

Ingredients:

- ½ teaspoon guar gum

- ½ teaspoon xanthan gum

- ½ teaspoon ocean salt

- ½ cup unsalted butter, cut into 3D squares

- 1 egg

- 1 tablespoon vinegar

- 1 tablespoon water

- 1 cup walnuts

- 1 cup almond flour, separated

- ⅔ cup ground brilliant flaxseeds

- 2 teaspoons baking powder

Directions:

1. In nourishment processor, beat the walnuts until slashed. Include ⅓ cup almond flour, the flaxseeds, baking powder, guar gum, xanthan gum, and salt. Beat until all around mixed.

2. Include the butter and heartbeat 10 times. Include the egg, vinegar, and water, and heartbeat until just consolidated. The mixture will be wet.

3. Dust a work surface and your hands with some almond dinner/flour.

4. Place the mixture on the work surface.

5. Massage the remaining almond supper into the mixture.

6. Structure into a plate. Wrap the mixture with plastic wrap.

7. Refrigerate for no less than 60 minutes. To take off, dust a piece of material paper with almond dinner.

8. Place the mixture on the paper and dust with more almond feast.

9. Top with a second piece of paper. With a rolling pin, move to a 10" round. Peel off the top paper.

10. Place a 9" pie plate upside down over the batter and turn the mixture onto the pie plate.

11. Tenderly peel off the material paper. Trim any shade and crease the edges.

12. Chill until prepared to use. To prebake, preheat the oven to 350°F.

13. Heat for 23 minutes, or until the crust is golden brown and no longer moist to touch.

Meatballs With Tomato Sauce

Ingredients:

- 1/3 cup whole wheat bread crumbs

- 12 oz. or 3 pieces sausages removed from casings

- 1 lb. ground beef (choose one with less fat)

- 1 tsp. minced garlic

- Salt

- ¼ cup Parmesan cheese

- 2 lightly beaten eggs

- Pepper

- Parmesan cheese for garnish

Sauce:

- 1 tbsp. minced garlic

- 2 cans tomatoes, diced and pureed

- 1 tsp. dried oregano

- 2 tsp. dried basil

- salt

Directions:

1. Preheat the oven to 425° F. Remove the sausages and ground beef from the cold.
2. Squeeze the sausage meat from their casings and bring both meats to room temperature.
3. Put the bread crumbs in a bowl and add 1/3 cup of hot water.
4. Let the crumbs absorb the water before adding the garlic, salt, pepper, grated Parmesan cheese and the eggs.
5. After mixing them well, add the meats and use your hands to combine them.

6. Prepare the pan or dish with oil or nonstick spray.

7. Round up meatballs with your hands, using a spoon to measure out the meat. Arrange them so they'll have space between each meatball.

8. Puree the tomatoes. After putting it in a bowl, add in the salt, herbs and garlic. Pour this sauce over the meatballs.

9. Sprinkle the remaining cheese over them. Bake them until the sauce and the cheese is bubbling. That would take just over half an hour.

10. Serve it hot with more Parmesan sprinkled on the meatballs.

Ham And Egg Breakfast Meal

Ingredients:

- 4 large eggs

- 8 slices of black forest ham

- Salt and ground pepper (salt is
  recommended to be coarse)

- Fresh chives, chopped into bits

Directions:

1. Preheat oven to 350° F. Prepare the pan and
   baking sheet with the olive oil.

2. Place four pieces of the ham on the baking
   pan and fold them in such a way that they
   have a "basket," folding the edges towards
   the center.

3. Crack an egg on each of the "basket" (you can
   use a muffin pan to make your life easier with

the hams), and cover with bits of the remaining ham.

4. Season with salt and pepper, then bake until the egg white has set, but with the yolk still runny.

5. That would take about 12 minutes.

6. Top with the chopped chives and serve hot.

Delicious Shrimp Bisque

Ingredients:

- ¾ pound peeled and deveined medium shrimp

- 1 cup tomato puree

- 1 tablespoon minced crisp parsley

- 2 teaspoons minced crisp dill

- 1 teaspoon lemon juice

- 2 cups chicken or vegetable juices

- 2 tablespoons butter or additional virgin olive oil

- 1 medium onion, slashed

- 1½ cups creamer or canned coconut milk

- Dash of ground red pepper

Directions:

1. In a medium pan over medium warmth, warm the butter or oil.

2. Cook the onion for 5 minutes, or until delicate. Include the shrimp, tomato puree, parsley, dill, lemon juice, and soup.

3. Stew for 10 minutes. Include the cream or coconut milk and the pepper and warmth through.

4. Serve embellished with the chive.

Chicken And Wild Rice Soup

Ingredients:

- 1 little onion, slashed

- 2 teaspoons lemon-pepper flavouring

- ½ teaspoon ocean salt

- 2 stalks broccoli, cut into little florets (2 cups)

- 2 cups creamer

- 6 cups chicken puree

- ½ cup wild rice

- 1 pound boneless, skinless chicken breasts, cubed

- 2 medium carrots, slashed

Directions:

1. In a vast pot over medium-high warmth, consolidate the chicken puree and rice.

2. Cover and convey to a boil. Decrease the warmth to medium-low and cook for 20 minutes. Include the chicken, carrots, onion, lemon-pepper flavouring, and salt. Cook for 15 minutes.

3. Include the broccoli and cook for 5 minutes, or until the broccoli and rice is delicate. Continuously mix in the creamer.

4. Cook, mixing, for 5 minutes, or until delicate. Serve while hot.

Chicken And Dumplings

Ingredients:

- 3 cups chicken puree

- 1 teaspoon dried thyme

- 1 pack Basic Biscuits (wheat free)

- ½ container harsh cream or canned coconut milk

- 2 tablespoons spread or coconut oil, isolated

- 8 boneless, skinless chicken thighs

- 2 onions, cleaved

- 2 carrots, cut 2 ribs

- celery, cut

Directions:

1. Preheat the oven to 350°F.
2. In a Dutch oven over medium-high warmth, warm 1 tablespoon of the margarine or oil.
3. Cook the chicken, turning sometimes, for 5 minutes, or until brilliant on all sides. Evacuate to a plate and put aside.
4. Heat the remaining 1 tablespoon spread or oil.
5. Cook the onions, carrots, and celery, blending sometimes, for 5 minutes, or until the onions begin to relax. Include the chicken puree, thyme, the remaining ⅛ teaspoon salt, and the held chicken.
6. Expand the warmth to high. Heat to the point of boiling. Heat, uncovered, for 20 minutes.
7. Meanwhile, prepare biscuits. Take out the Dutch oven from the oven and stir in the sour cream or coconut milk.
8. Increase the oven temperature to 400°F. Dollop 8 biscuits into the chicken mixture.

9. Bake for 15 minutes, uncovered.

10. Cover and bake for 15 minutes, or until a thermometer inserted in the deepest part of the chicken registers 170°F.

Homemade Granola Bar

Ingredients:

- 1 cup macadamia nuts

- 1 tbsp. vanilla concentrate

- ½ tsp. cinnamon

- 2 cup almonds

- 1 cup pumpkin seeds

- 1 cup raisins

- Salt

Directions:

1. On a substantial dish, drench the almonds, macadamia nuts, and pumpkin seeds overnight.

2. Do likewise with the raisins on another dish. Puree the raisins on a blender or nourishment processor, including the drenching water.

3. In the meantime, strain and wash the nuts from their splashing water.

4. Blend in the nuts onto the raisin puree and mix a couple of times until coming to your coveted consistency or composition.

5. Include vanilla, cinnamon and salt, then mix together.

6. Empty the mixture into a preparing sheet then prepare in the oven for around 45 minutes at 250 degrees.

Trail Mix Snacks

Ingredients:

- 1 cup raisins

- 1 cup almonds

- 3 cup dried cranberries

- 3 cup macadamia nuts

Directions:

1. Basically blend and hurl all the fixings together in an extensive large bowl.

2. Store in glass containers or any favoured holder. Serve when peckish diminishes.

Spicy Party Mix Wheat Free Snacks

Ingredients:

- 1 cup brilliant raisins

- 3 tbsp. bean stew powder

- 1 tsp. chipotle powder

- 1 cup crude cashews

- 1 cup cut almonds

- 1 cup pecans

Directions:

1. Hurl the nuts (cashews, almonds, pecans) with the olive oil in a dish.

2. Season with the bean stew and chipotle powder and the ocean salt with consistent hurling.

3. Spread uniformly on a treat sheet lined with material paper.

4. Place in an oven for ten minutes at most more than 350 degrees.
5. When evacuated, let the blend cool before hurling in the raisins and serve instantly.

Onion, Garlic & Kale

Ingredients:

- 3 tbsp olive oil

- 1 onion, chopped

- 3 bunches kale - washed, dried, and shredded

- 3 cloves garlic, minced

- 1 cup bread crumbs

Directions:

1. Warm 1tbsp of olive oil over high heat in a non-stick skillet. Toss in the garlic and onion.

2. Cook for 5-7 minutes or until both the garlic and onion have softened.

3. Toss in the breadcrumbs and mix to incorporate. Cook for 2-3 minutes or until the breadcrumbs have browned.

4. Throw in the kale and cook for another 2-3 minutes, or until the kale has wilted.

5. Stir throughout to ensure the vegetables do not burn.

Quinoa & Black Beans

Ingredients:

- 1 tsp ground cumin

- 1 tbsp sunflower oil

- 1 onion, chopped

- 4 cloves garlic, chopped

- ½ tsp cayenne pepper

- A pinch of salt & pepper

- 1 cup frozen corn kernels

- 2* 14oz canned black beans, rinsed and drained

- 1 ½ cups vegetable broth

- 1 cup quinoa

Directions:

1. In a medium saucepan, warm 1 tbsp sunflower oil.

2. Toss in the garlic and onion and cook for 5-7 minutes or until both vegetables have softened.

3. Combine quinoa with the onion and garlic, stirring to ensure an even distribution.

4. Add the vegetable broth and throw in all the seasonings except the cilantro.

5. Cover the saucepan and lower the heat until a gentle simmer is produced. Cook for 20 minutes.

6. Toss in the corn and cook for 5 minutes. Finally, throw in the cilantro and the black beans.

7. Heat for a moment or two to ensure the beans are warm. Serve immediately.

Chocolate Dipped Walnut And Currant Cookies

Ingredients:

- 1 cup pecans

- 6 tbsp coconut palm sugar

- ¼ tsp ground cinnamin'1/2 cup currants

- 1 tsp pure vanilla extract

- 3 cups chopped walnuts

- ½ cup almond flour

- 1/3 tsp pure stevia extract

- 1/8 tsp sea salt

- 2 whisked eggs

For dipping

- ½ tsp coconut oil

- 4 oz dark or semisweet chocolate

Directions:

1. Preheat the oven to 350 degrees.
2. Line the baking sheet with parchment paper then set aside.
3. Process the walnuts and pecans until it has the same texture as a meal. Continue to pulse until the mixture clumps together.
4. Add the nut mixture to a medium bowl and combine with the almond flour, cinnamon, salt and sweetener. Mix to combine.
5. Stir in the currants, vanilla and egg until you have dough.
6. Scoop the batter and shape into balls. Flatten the dough ball slightly.
7. Bake for 15 minutes until the edges are golden and slightly firm.
8. Remove from the oven and place on a rack to cool.

9. Heat the coconut oil and chocolate in a broiler until it is fully melted. Dip one side of the cookies in the chocolate and place on the parchment paper.

10. Sprinkle with powdered sugar if desired.

11. Place in the refrigerator to harden.

Gingerbread People

Ingredients:

- 1 egg

- 3 cups almond flour

- 1 tsp ground ginger

- ½ tsp cinnamon

- 1 tsp baking soda

- 8 tbsp butter or coconut oil

- 1/3 cup honey

- ½ tsp allspice

- ½ tsp ground cloves

- 1/8 tsp sea salt

Directions:

1. Combine the salt, flour, spice and baking soda together in a bowl.

2. Add the rest of the ingredients. Stir it until the dough is formed.

3. Form one large dough or two medium sized balls.

4. Freeze in the refrigerator for 30 minutes.

5. Preheat the oven at 350 degrees.

6. Place parchment paper above and below the dough to prevent it from sticking.

7. Spread some almond flour below the dough.

8. Roll and shape the cookies.

9. Gently place the cookies on the baking sheet.

10. Bake for 10 minutes until the edges are brown.

11. Place in a warm oven for 20 minutes.

12. Allow to cool before decorating.

Asparagus Frittata

Ingredients:

- ½ tsp salt

- 2 tbsp unsalted butter

- 1/3 cup minced shallots

- 6 large eggs

- 1 cup shredded Swiss cheese

- 1 lb asparagus, cut diagonally into 1 inch lengths

Directions:

1. Heat the butter in a frying pan over medium heat.
2. Cook the shallots and stir occasionally for about 3 minutes.
3. Add in the asparagus and cover for another 3 minutes. Pour in eggs until almost set.

4. Sprinkle cheese then cook for 6 minutes.

5. Remove from heat then serve.

Baby Bok Choy With Cashews

Ingredients:

- 1 lb baby bok choy, rinsed and separated

- ½ tsp sesame oil

- ½ cup salted cashews

- 2 tbsp olive oil

- 3 garlic cloves

- Salt

Directions:

1. Heat the oil in a pan then add the onions, garlic and bok choy.
2. Season it with sesame oil and salt.
3. Cook for 3 minutes. Gently add the cashews then simmer.

Baked Beans In Tomato Sauce

Ingredients:

- 1 tsp chili flakes

- ½ onion chopped

- 2 tbsp honey

- ¼ cup tomato paste

- 15 oz tomato sauce

- 2 cups chicken broth

- 1 lb dry cannellini

- 1 tbsp olive oil

- ¼ lb bacon finely chopped

- 4 chopped garlic

- 1 tbsp minced sage

- 1/2 cup chopped parsley

- 2 tbsp balsamic vinegar

- Salt and pepper to taste

Directions:

1. Soak the beans in water overnight.
2. Drain the beans and put them in a pot then cover with water.
3. Bring to a simmer then lower the heat until the beans are soft enough. Preheat the oven to 325 degrees.
4. In a pot, heat the olive oil and add the bacon and cook.
5. Mix in the onions and stir until the onion begins to brown.
6. Add garlic, chili flakes, honey, tomato paste and sage. Stir well to combine.
7. Bring to a simmer then season with salt and pepper.

8. Sprinkle with chopped parsley and vinegar.

Vegetable Stir-Fry

Ingredients:

- ½ tray sugar snap peas

- 1 pc small ginger, chopped

- ½ clove garlic, crushed

- 1 tsp coconut butter

- ¾ tsp Tamari sauce

- ½ head broccoli, chopped

- ½ pc fennel, sliced

- 1 pc courgette, sliced

- Some coriander, chopped

Directions:

1. Fry ginger and garlic on coconut butter until lightly brown.
2. Add broccoli, fennel, courgette and sugar snap peas.
3. Add Tamari sauce and a little water. Fry while stirring and letting the vegetable steam through.
4. Remove from fire, top with chopped coriander as garnishing.
5. Serve with rice. This makes 3-4 servings.

Chicken With Prunes And Green Olives

Ingredients:

- 1 cup chicken broth, low to no salt

- ¼ cup red wine vinegar

- ¼ cup green olives, pitted and chopped

- ¼ cup prunes or dried plums, pitted and chopped

- 1 pc ¼-pound chicken thighs, trimmed of fat, deboned and skinned

- 1 tsp extra virgin olive oil

- Ground pepper to taste

Directions:

1. Clean and rinse chicken, and pat dry with a paper towel.
2. Heat olive oil in a large nonstick pan or skillet over medium to high heat.
3. Cook chicken in oil, 2 minutes per side, until brown.
4. Add chicken broth and vinegar, and bring to a simmer while stirring constantly.
5. Add olives, prunes and some pepper. Put heat to low.
6. Cook for 12 to 15 minutes, or until chicken is no longer pink in the middle.
7. Transfer chicken to a large plate, and serve. This makes 4 servings.
8. Meats such as beef, pork, chicken, fish, and other types of seafood, are generally wheat-free.
9. Avoid adding breading to them, since most breading mixes contain flour or wheat.

10. The same is true for processed meat products such as burger patties, hotdogs, and sausages.

11. Other easy and quick to prepare options: steamed carrots, steamed green beans, baked sweet potato, steamed broccoli spears, and steamed cauliflower.

Mushroom Frittata With Broccoli

Ingredients:

- 2 cups broccoli florets

- 1 teaspoon ocean salt

- ½ teaspoon ground black pepper

- 1 cup destroyed sharp Cheddar cheese

- 2 cups cream

- 6 eggs

- 1 clove garlic, daintily cut

- 1 teaspoon additional virgin olive oil

- 8 ounces cremini mushrooms, cut

- 2 tablespoons approximately pressed new dill, slashed

Directions:

1. Preheat the oven to 375°F. Oil a 9" pie plate. In a little skillet, cook the garlic in the oil over medium-low warmth for 3 minutes.

2. Evacuate the garlic and put aside. Build the warmth to medium.

3. Cook the mushrooms, blending habitually, for 8 minutes, or until brilliant.

4. In the interim, put a steamer wicker bin in an expansive pot with 2" of water over medium-high heat.

5. Steam the broccoli for 3 minutes, or until brilliant green and delicate fresh. Remove what's more and generally slash.

6. Add the broccoli to the skillet. Mix to coat. Sprinkle with salt and pepper.

7. Expel from the warmth, and include the saved garlic.

8. Line the base of the pie plate with the vegetables. Top with the cheese.

9. In a dish, whisk together the cream and eggs.

10. Add the dill and race to join. Deliberately pour over the cheese and vegetables.

11. Place the pie plate on a baking sheet and prepare in the focal point of the oven for 35 minutes, or until a knife embedded in the middle comes out clean.

Mushroom Frittata With Artichokes

Ingredients:

- 1/ 3 cup water

- 1 little clove garlic, slashed finely

- 2 medium unfenced eggs

- 1 ½ tablespoons feta cheese, disintegrated

- 1 ½-ounces (around 2 tablespoons) mushrooms, cut daintily

- 1 tablespoon of additional virgin coconut oil, partitioned

- 2 infant artichokes, trimmed and divided Flakes

- ocean salt and black pepper, to taste

Directions:

1. In a pan, warm 1 tablespoon of oil on medium-high warmth. Include artichokes. Sprinkle a squeeze of salt and black pepper.

2. Sauté for around 3 to 4 minutes. Decrease the warmth to medium-low. Include water and garlic.

3. Cover and stew for around 10 minutes. Uncover and cook until all water is consumed.

4. Expel from stove. Dry the artichokes with a paper towel.

5. Leave any abundance oil in the skillet. Preheat the oven. In a dish, include eggs, ½ tablespoon of cheese and squeeze of salt and black pepper and beat until very much consolidated.

6. In a skillet, warmth remaining oil (or include ½ tablespoon coconut oil if essential) on medium-high warmth. Include mushrooms

and sauté for around 3 to 4 minutes or until chestnut.

7. Add sautéed artichokes and keep on cooking, mixing for around 2 minutes. Mix in eggs.

8. Decrease the warmth to medium.

9. Cover and cook for around 3 to 4 minutes or until eggs are situated. Sprinkle remaining cheese on top.

10. Presently, put the skillet in oven. Sear for around 1 minute. Serve this frittata with a plate of mixed green salad.

Parmesan Cheese Soufflé

Ingredients:

- 1 cup milk, at room temperature

- ½ teaspoon fine ocean salt

- ¼ teaspoon ground black pepper

- ¼ teaspoon nutmeg

- 4 tablespoons butter, liquefied and separated

- 2 tablespoons ground Parmesan cheese

- 4 eggs + 1 egg yolk

- 3 tablespoons garbanzo bean (chickpea) flour

Directions:

1. Preheat the oven to 425° F. Brush six 6-ounce ramekins with 2 tablespoons softened butter, furthermore, tidy with the cheese.

2. Place on a baking sheet and put aside.

3. Separate the eggs, putting the yolks in a medium dish and the whites in an expansive dish.

4. In a medium saucepan over medium warmth, dissolve the remaining 2 tablespoons butter.

5. Include the flour and cook, whisking continually, for 1 to 2 minutes, or until mixed and the mixture starts to air pocket.

6. Slowly include the milk, whisking always until smooth.

7. Cook, whisking always, for 5 minutes, or until the mixture starts to thicken.

8. Try not to let the mixture boil. Expel from the warmth and include the salt, pepper, and nutmeg.

9. Whisking continually, pour ⅓ cup of the milk mixture into the yolks.

10. At that point include the remaining milk mixture to the dish and whisk altogether.

11. On the off chance that setting up the soufflé the night before serving it, cover the yolk mixture and the egg whites and refrigerate both overnight.

12. Permit both to come to room temperature (enough to take the chill off) some time recently continuing.

13. With an electric mixer on rapid, beat the egg whites until delicate crests structure.

14. Fold 33% of the egg whites into the yolk mixture. Rehash.

15. Isolate the mixture into the ramekins. Prepare in the focal point of the oven for 17 to 18 minutes, then again until puffed and brilliant.

16. The focuses ought to look set and firm, and a toothpick embedded into the inside ought to tell the truth out. Serve while hot.

Onion Rings

Ingredients:

- ½ red pepper powder or chili powder

- 1 tsp. ground black pepper

- Salt

- 250 ml beer

- 2 onions, choose the white ones

- ¼ cup almond meal with some more for "breading" the onion rings

Directions:

1. Mix the almond meal, red and black pepper, salt and beer.
2. Make sure all the ingredients are mixed evenly.
3. Afterwards, cover it and let it sit for an hour.
4. In a pan, heat about 5 cm-high peanut or olive oil until it is around 370° F.
5. On a plate filled with some almond meal, toss 5 or 6 pieces of onion rings, and then dip it in your prepared batter. Drop them one at a time into the oil.
6. Cook the rings for a few minutes until they are sufficiently browned on both sides.
7. Drain off all oil with paper towels or by putting them on a wire rack. Salt the rings and serve hot.

Eggplant-Veggie Snacks

Ingredients:

- 1 cup spaghetti sauce or tomato sauce of your choice

- 1 eggplant (1 ¼ lbs.)

- Seasoning of your choice

- ½ cup beaten eggs

- ¾ tsp. garlic and salt powder

Directions:

1. Cut eggplant into snack-sized sticks.
2. In a long bowl or on a dish, combine the garlic and salt powder, with your choice seasoning. Dip each eggplant stick into the beaten eggs then coat it in the powder mixture. Arrange them on a baking sheet.
3. Spray the laid out sticks with cooking spray. Broil the sticks for 3 minutes.

4. Remove the baking sheet from the oven afterwards.

5. Turn the sticks and spritz them again with the cooking spray.

6. Cook for another 2 minutes or when they are browned to your liking.

7. Serve hot. Prepare the tomato sauce as your dip. Or any other dip you have decided to prepare.

Delicious Fish Sticks

Ingredients:

- 6 tbsp. Olive oil

- 1 cup almond flour

- 1/2 kg. White fish fillet

- 2 eggs

- Salt

Directions:

1. Flush the cuts of fish and place on a plate. Uproot the bones of the fish and cut into 1 by 5 inch rectangles.
2. Blend the flour and salt in one bowl, the eggs in a different dish.
3. Dunk the fish into the eggs in the first place, then into the flour rapidly. Set up all the fish in this way on a plate.

4. Over medium warmth, warm a pan with three tablespoons of olive oil.
5. Place 50% of the fish fillets on the pan sufficiently leaving space to turn them over and cook.
6. Cook every side of the fish until chestnut. Serve with your favourite sauce or ketchup.

Tasty Creamy Parmesan Chicken

Ingredients:

- 1 can (13.6 ounces) coconut milk

- 1 cup destroyed Gouda, Swiss, or Colby cheese

- ½ cup ground Parmesan cheese, isolated

- 4 boneless, skinless chicken breast parts

- 6 scallions, white and light green parts, meagrely cut

Directions:

1. Preheat the oven to 375°F. Coat a 9" × 9" heating dish with cooking shower.

2. Place the chicken in the dish. Sprinkle with the scallions. In a medium dish, join the coconut

milk, Gouda, Swiss, or Colby, and ¼ cup of the Parmesan.

3. Pour over the chicken mixture. Sprinkle with the remaining ¼ cup Parmesan.

4. Heat for 30 minutes, or until percolating and a thermometer embedded in the thickest segment registers 165°F and the juices run clear. Let stand for 5 minutes prior to serving.

Glazed Pork Tenderloin

Ingredients:

- ¼ teaspoon ocean salt

- 2 tablespoons coconut oil, additional virgin olive oil, or butter

- ¼ cup beef puree

- 1 tablespoon balsamic vinegar

- 2 tablespoons Dijon mustard

- 1 pound pork tenderloin

- 1 teaspoon ground cardamom

- ½ teaspoon ground dark pepper

Directions:

1. Preheat the oven to 350°F.

2. On a work surface, rub the tenderloin uniformly with the cardamom, pepper, and

salt. In a heatproof heating pan or oven proof skillet over medium-high warmth, warm the oil.

3. Cook the tenderloin, turning at times, for 8 minutes, or until sautéed on all sides.

4. Place in the oven. Cook for 20 minutes, or until a thermometer embedded in the middle registers 160°F and the juices run clear.

5. Expel from the oven and exchange the pork to a cutting board. Let stand for 10 minutes.

6. Place the skillet over medium-high warmth.

7. Include the beef puree and vinegar. Heat to the point of boiling, mixing to uproot any cooked bits.

8. Cook until the mixture is decreased by about half. Rush in the mustard.

9. Cut the pork and shower with the sauce.

Beaded Pork Chops

Ingredients:

- 1 teaspoon sans gluten soy sauce

- ½ cup ground pecans

- 4 boneless pork loin slashes, ¾" thick

- 2 tablespoons olive or coconut oil

- 2 tablespoons ground brilliant flaxseeds

- ½ teaspoon ocean salt

- ½ teaspoon smoked paprika

- 1 vast egg

Directions:

1. On a plate, join the flaxseeds, salt, and paprika.

2. In a wide shallow dish, whisk the egg and soy sauce.

3. Place the pecans on a plate.

4. Dunk every hack into the flax mixture, then in the egg mixture, and after that into the pecans to coat.

5. In a huge skillet over medium-high warmth, warm the oil.

6. Cook the pork hacks for 8 minutes, turning once, or until a thermometer embedded sideways in a cleave registers 160°F and the juices run clear.

Glazed Salmon

Ingredients:

- 1 clove garlic, minced

- A pinch of garlic salt

- A pinch of pepper

- 1 lb salmon

- ¼ cup maple syrup

- 4 tsp soy sauce

Directions:

1. Preheat your oven to 400F.

2. Combine together the maple syrup, garlic, garlic salt, pepper and soy sauce.

3. Place the salmon on a baking dish and glaze it with the maple dressing previously made.

4. Bake for 20 minutes, or until the salmon disintegrates upon light pressure.

Vegetable Chili

Ingredients:

- 3 cloves garlic, chopped

- 2*4oz canned green chilli peppers, drained

- ¼ cup chilli powder

- 1 tsp ground cumin

- 2 tbsp dried oregano

- 1 tbsp ground black pepper

- 1*14oz canned kidney beans, drained

- 2*12 oz vegetarian burger crumbles

- 6*14oz canned chopped tomatoes

- 1*14oz canned garbanzo beans, drained

- 1*14oz canned black beans

- 3 tsp olive oil

- ½ medium onion, chopped

- 2 bay leaves

- 3 green bell peppers, chopped

- 2 jalapeno peppers, chopped

- 1 tbsp salt

- 1 stalks celery, chopped

Directions:

1. In a large saucepan, warm 3 tbsp of olive oil over a high heat.
2. Toss in the onion, garlic and bay leaves, oregano, cumin and a pinch of salt.

3. Cook for 5-7 minutes or until the onions have softened.

4. Next, add celery, green bell peppers , jalapeno peppers & green chilli peppers.

5. Cook for 10-15 minutes or until all the vegetables have softened. Stir continuously throughout to ensure nothing burns.

6. Next, add the vegetable burger protein. Lower the temperature until there is a mild simmer. Cover and leave to simmer gently for 5-7 minutes.

7. After this, add the chopped tomatoes to the saucepan, alongside the chilli powder, pepper and beans.

8. Raise the heat and bring the content of the pan to a boil.

9. Cover, reduce the heat and cook for 45 minutes.

10. Remove the lid and add the corn. Cook for 5 more minutes. Finally serve immediately.

Toffee Almond Flour Cookies

Ingredients:

- ½ cup sugar

- 1 tsp vanilla extract

- ½ tsp baking soda

- ¾ cup toffee bits

- ½ cup softened butter

- 1 egg

- ½ tsp salt

- 3 cups almond flour

Directions:

1. Preheat the oven to 375 degrees.

2. Cream the sugar and butter for 3 minutes.

3. Add the egg and vanilla. Beat the mixture until the ingredients are well incorporated. Add this to the almond mixture.

4. Add the baking soda and salt and stir together. Add to the almond mixture.

5. Gently add toffee bits.

6. Scoop about one and one half tablespoon of the mixture into the baking sheet. You can also use an ice cream scooper to transfer the mixture to the baking sheet.

7. Smooth out the dough to make the cookies.

8. Bake for 10 minutes at 375 degrees.

9. Allow to cool for 5 minutes before serving.

Peanut Butter Almond Flour Cookies

Ingredients:

- 1 tsp vanilla extract

- ¼ cup sugar

- ½ tsp salt

- 1/3 cup peanut butter

- ½ cup almond flour

- ½ tsp baking soda

- 1 egg

Directions:

1. Preheat the oven.
2. Combine the sugar, baking soda, salt and almond flour.
3. Beat the egg, peanut butter and vanilla.

4. Gently add the wet ingredients to the mix using your hands.
5. Divide the mixture in half and repeat the process until you have 8 sections.
6. Roll each section into dough. Use a fork to push the cookie down and make a cross pattern.
7. Bake the cookies for 11 minutes.
8. Place on the cooling tray for half an hour before serving.

Chicken Marbella

Ingredients:

- ½ cup pitted prunes

- 8 large green olives

- ¼ cup brown sugar

- ½ cup white wine

- 2 tbsp Italian parsley

- 3 bay leaves

- 2 chickens

- ½ cup garlic

- 2 tbsp dried oregano

- ¼ cup red wine vinegar

- ¼ cup olive oil

Directions:

1. Combine garlic, oregano, olive oil, bay leaves, prunes, olives, capers and caper juice in a large bowl. Add the chicken and marinate overnight.
2. Preheat the oven to 350 degrees.
3. Arrange the chicken in a baking pan and spoon marinade over it. Bake for 50 minutes.
4. Transfer to a platter and sprinkle with parsley and cilantro.

Chipotle Lime Bacon-Wrapped Shrimp

Ingredients:

- Zest from 1 lime

- ¼ tsp chipotle powder

- 6 strips of bacon

- 12 large peeled shrimps

- 2 tbsp olive oil

- Juice from 1 lime

Directions:

1. Mix the lime zest and juice with chipotle powder and olive oil.
2. Place the shrimp in the mixture and make sure everything is coated.
3. Spread the bacon in a microwave-safe oven.
4. Bake until the bacon fat begins to melt.

5. Wrap bacon around a shrimp and thread into skewers or bamboo sticks.

6. Brush lime chipotle into the shrimp and bake or grill.

Banana-Raspberry With Coconut Milk And Sunflower Seeds

Ingredients:

- 1 cup fresh raspberries

- 1 tbsp sunflower seeds

- 1 pc large ripe banana, sliced

- ½ cup coconut milk

Directions:

1. In a bowl, place sliced banana and top with creamy coconut milk.
2. Add raspberries and sunflower seeds. Lightly toss. This makes 1 to 2 servings.

Quinoa-Orange Porridge

Ingredients:

- ½ cup water

- 1 pc fresh orange, peeled and chopped.

- 50g quinoa

- ½ cup rice milk

Directions:

1. Mix rice milk and water in saucepan set over low to medium fire.
2. Add quinoa and bring to a boil. Let it simmer until tender, or until all the liquid has been fully absorbed.
3. Remove from fire. Stir in chopped oranges and serve in a bowl. This makes 2-3 servings.

Mixed Berries With Yogurt And Pumpkin Seeds

Ingredients:

- 200g natural live yogurt (or Greek yogurt, or plain, unsweetened yogurt)

- 1 tbsp pumpkin seeds

- 200g berries (any type), fresh (if frozen or tinned, choose unsweetened ones)

Directions:

1. Place all ingredients in a blender, and blend thoroughly.
2. To round up your breakfast, try adding a piece or slice of any fruit.
3. You may also drink milk or add some cheese since they do not contain any wheat.

4. Check the labels, though, since some types of cottage cheese may contain wheat fillers.

5. Be careful of the type of milk, since there are flavored ones that contain wheat, such as malted milk.

6. If you are to add eggs to your breakfast, it would be better to consume them in the usual manners: scrambled, fried, or hard-boiled. If you try making quiche or soufflés, it is more than likely that you will have to use other ingredients that contain wheat.

7. THIS IS IMPORTANT: when preparing meals, make sure that the ingredients do not come into contact with other ingredients that contain wheat. This is to prevent contamination.

8. Therefore, see to it that you have separate tools or utensils for preparing regular meals (for those who are not following the wheat-free diet) and for preparing wheat-free meals.

Green Chile Strata

Ingredients:

- 4 eggs

- 2 cups milk

- 1 teaspoon ocean salt

- ½ teaspoon ground black pepper

- 1 teaspoon cumin

- 2½ cups destroyed Monterey Jack cheese, separated

- 2 links chorizo (around 7 ounces), housings uprooted

- ½ little onion, finely hacked

- 1 Serrano chile pepper, seeded and finely hacked

- ½ chunk Basic Bread (page 225), cut into ½" blocks (around 4 cups)

- Oil a 9" × 9" baking pan.

Directions:

1. Heat a medium skillet over medium-high warmth.
2. Cook the chorizo, breaking with a wooden spoon, for 5 minutes. Lessen the warmth to medium and include the onion and chile pepper.
3. Cook, blending once in a while, for 8 minutes, or until the chorizo is cooked through and the vegetables are diminished.
4. Exchange to a plate secured with a paper towel and put aside to cool marginally.
5. In a substantial dish, whisk together the eggs, milk, salt, black pepper, and cumin.
6. Blend in 2 cups of the cheese, the bread blocks, and the chorizo mixture until consolidated. Fill the baking pan.

7. Cover and refrigerate for 8 hours or overnight.

8. To prepare, preheat the oven to 375° F. Uncover the strata and top with the remaining ½ cup cheese.

9. Prepare for 35 minutes, or until puffed and a knife comes out clean when inserted.

Green Pepper Omelet With Spinach

Ingredients:

- Flaked ocean salt, to taste

- Black pepper powder, to taste

- Cayenne pepper, to taste

- 2 tablespoons water

- 4 free roaming eggs

- 2 tablespoons parmesan cheese, destroyed

- 3 teaspoons additional virgin coconut oil, partitioned

- ½ cup green bell pepper, seeded, roasted, evacuate seeds and black skin and cut into slim strips

- ¾ cup spinach, stemmed and torn

Directions:

1. In a non-stick skillet, include 2 teaspoons of oil and bell pepper and simply warm for around 1 moment.

2. Include spinach and cook until simply shriveled for around 30 to 40 seconds. Expel from the pan and move into a dish.

3. Sprinkle a little squeeze of salt, black pepper and cayenne pepper.

4. In another dish, include water, eggs, squeeze of salt and black pepper and beat until very much consolidated.

5. Coat a non-stick griddle with remaining oil. Heat the pan on medium warmth. Include the beaten eggs in pan and diminish the warmth to medium-low.

6. Cook, without blending for around 2 minutes.

7. Place the spinach mixture in the inside. Sprinkle the cheese over spinach mixture.

8. At that point roll the omelet and spot into a serving plate. Serve this omelet with avocado slices.

Sausage Bits Snack

Ingredients:

- 12 oz. pork sausages, ground

- Ham slices

- Scrambled eggs, fried

- 12 oz. spicy pork sausages, ground

- mayonnaise

Directions:

1. Preheat your broiler.

2. Mix and cook the ground pork sausage and the spicy ground pork sausage in a well-oiled skillet.

3. Brown the ground pork over medium high heat. Drain the sausage of any liquid.

4. Process the ground pork with the mayonnaise until they are incorporated well.

5. On each ham slice, place some of the ground pork mixture and some scrambled eggs.

6. Roll them up and secure with a toothpick.

7. Broil the rolls for 3 to 5 minutes.

8. Check it frequently, and finishing when they are sufficiently toasted.

Chickpeas Snack

Ingredients:

- 1 tsp. coriander

- 1 tsp. cumin

- 1 tsp. garlic powder

- 1 tsp. curry powder

- Olive oil or cooking spray

- Salt

- 1 tsp. chili powder

- 1 tsp. paprika

Directions:

1. Preheat oven to 375° F. Drain chickpeas and let them completely dry.

2. If you need to, you can pat dry them with a paper towel.

3. Arrange them on a baking sheet, laying them on a single layer.

4. Roast for around half an hour, shaking the pan every ten minutes. Just make sure they don't burn.

5. You'll know they are done when they have turned golden brown with crunchy insides, instead of moist.

6. Combine all the spices in a bowl, mixing them well. Remove the chickpeas from the oven when they are done and spray them with olive oil.

7. Toss the chickpeas with the spices while they're still hot.

8. They are preferably served hot. But you can also let them cool in room temperature and then place them in airtight plastic zip bags afterwards.

Coco-Nutty, Limey, Grilled Pineapples

Ingredients:

- 2 tbsp. toasted coconut bits

- 3 slices of pineapples, can be ring or strips, 2 inches thick

- 1 lime, cut into wedges

Directions:

1. Heat the grill (or the pan if you're using one).
2. Grill the pineapples. Stop when the fruits are getting caramelized. Transfer into a plate.
3. Garnish with the lime wedges and sprinkle some coconut bits on top.

Sweet Peach Crisp

Ingredients:

- ½ tsp. vanilla concentrate

- 2 tbsp. Butter

- 1 ¼ c. almond flour, whitened

- 1 kg. peaches, cut

- 1 tbsp. maple syrup

- Salt

Directions:

1. Lay out the cut peaches into a heating dish.
2. Blend the almond flour and salt in a sustenance processor.
3. At that point, beat with the butter, maple syrup, and vanilla.
4. Pour mixture over the peaches. Prepare in the oven for roughly 45 minutes at 350 degrees.

5. Give it a chance to cool before serving.

Sweet Macaroons

Ingredients:

- ¼ cup nectar

- 2 tbsp. additional virgin coconut oil

- 1 tbsp. vanilla concentrate

- 1 ½ cup destroyed coconut, unsweetened

- 1 tbsp. coconut flour

- salt

Directions:

1. Blend the destroyed coconuts with the coconut flour in the nourishment processor. Join with nectar, coconut oil, salt, and vanilla concentrate by beating.

2. Shape mixture into a ball. Spot balls into a preparing sheet for heating.

3. For a most extreme of 7 minutes, bake at 350 degrees.

4. Let the macaroons cool for two or three hours prior to serving.

Pineapple Tapioca

Ingredients:

- Tapioca, 1 cup.

- Pineapple juice, 1 cup.

- Water, 4 cups.

- Sugar, 2-3 cup.

Directions:

1. Better results take after when the tapioca is splashed over night or for a few hours.
2. Wash the tapioca, and splash in the water; just before cooking include sugar and pineapple juice.
3. Cook in a twofold boiler until straightforward, and pour into a level dish to cool.
4. On the off chance that cut pineapple is within reach, dice it, and place in the base of the dish, before pouring in the tapioca.

5. On the off chance that, when cooking tapioca or sago for pudding, it ought to cook too long and get flimsy, it might be made into a decent pastry by beating it into beaten egg whites; season, and shape in cups or dish. Present with a hued sauce.

Cheese Fondue

Ingredients:

- ½ teaspoon dry mustard

- 1 clove garlic, divided

- 1 cup chicken puree

- 3 ounces cream cheese, cut into lumps

- 2 cups destroyed Gruyère cheese (8 ounces)

- 2 cups destroyed Swiss cheese (8 ounces)

- 1 tablespoon arrowroot

Directions:

1. In a medium dish, hurl the Gruyere and Swiss with the arrowroot and mustard until covered.
2. Rub the garlic parts all around within the highest point of a twofold boiler, and then toss.
3. Add the chicken puree to the twofold boiler and place over stewing water.
4. Step by step include the cheese mixture, blending until the cheeses are dissolved.
5. Mix in the cream cheese just until softened.
6. Expel from the warmth. Keep warm in a fondue pot while serving.

Garlic & Bay Tilapia

Ingredients:

- 1 tsp garlic salt

- 1 lemon, sliced

- 16oz mixed frozen broccoli & cauliflower

- 4*4oz fillets tilapia

- 1 tbsp butter

- A pinch of Old Bay Seasoning

Directions:

1. Preheat the oven to 375F. Use low-calories cooking spray to grease a 9*13 baking dish.
2. Place the butter and tilapia fillets in the baking dish. Sprinkle with old bay seasoning and garlic salt.

3. Next, place each tilapia fillet with a slice or lemon.

4. Fill the rest of the baking dish with the frozen cauliflower and broccoli.

5. Dust the entire mixture with a pinch of salt and pepper.

6. Roast for 30 minutes, or until all vegetables are tender and the fish breaks upon slight pressure.

Strawberry & Banana Smoothie

Ingredients:

- ½ tsp vanilla extract

- 2 tsp caster sugar

- 1 banana, roughly chopped

- 15 frozen strawberries

- 1 cup soy milk

- ¾ cup rolled oats

Directions:

1. Add all ingredients to a food blender and process in pulses. Pulse until smooth.
2. Separate into two serving glasses and serve immediately.

Shrimp Cake

Ingredients:

- 1 egg

- ½ cup blanched almond flour

- 1 red or yellow bell pepper, chopped

- 2 tbsp thinly sliced scallions

- 1 tbsp agave nectar

- ¼ tsp chipotle chili, ground

- ½ cup finely chopped cilantro

- 1 lb peeled and deveined shrimp

- 1 minced garlic clove

- 1 tbsp lime juice, freshly squeezed

- ½ tsp Celtic sea salt

- 3 tbsp grape seed oil

Directions:

1. Place the shrimp in a blender then process until it is finely chopped.
2. Mix the shrimp, scallions, agave, lime, garlic, bell pepper, salt, egg, chipotle and cilantro in a large bowl.
3. Form the mixture in thick patties and coat with the almond flour.
4. Pour one tablespoon of the oil in a large pan.
5. Add the patties to the pan and cook for about 5 minutes per side until it is brown.
6. Remove and place on top of paper towels.
7. Repeat the procedure with the rest of the cakes.

Cod Picasa

Ingredients:

- ¼ cup fresh chopped parsley

- ½ cup blanched almond flour

- ½ tsp all-purpose chef's shake

- 5 tbsp all olive oil

- 1 cup chicken stock

- ¼ cup brined capers

- 1 ½ lb cod

- ½ tsp Celtic sea salt

- 5 tbsp grape seed oil or butter

- ¼ cup lemon juice

Directions:

1. Chop the cod into 6 pieces.

2. Combine the salt, chef's shake and flour in a bowl.
3. Rinse the fish in cold water then dip into the flour mixture. Roll to coat.
4. Heat the oil in a pan over medium heat. Add half of the fish pieces and cook well for 3 minutes per side.
5. Transfer the fish to a plate. Cook the rest of the cod.
6. Place the plate of cod in the oven then start to prepare the sauce.
7. Add the lemon juice, stock and capers into the pan.
8. Scrape the brown bits at the bottom to incorporate it to the sauce.
9. Reduce the sauce by half then add the remaining grape seed oil.
10. Place in a plate then pour the sauce over then sprinkle with parsley.
11. Serve warm.

Chicken Parmesan

Ingredients:

- 1 tsp herbs de province

- 16 oz mozzarella cheese

- 2 cups blanched almond flour

- 6 tbsp salted butter

- 2 cups water

- 4 boneless and skinless chicken breast

- 2 eggs, whisked

- 7 oz tomato paste

- 6 sliced garlic cloves

Directions:

1. Slice the chicken in half to have thinner cutlets. Pat it dry then set aside.

2. Dip the chicken in egg and allow the excess to drain.

3. Coat it with the almond flour.

4. Melt the butter in a pan then cook the chicken until it is golden brown on both sides.

5. Place the chicken on a paper towel to drain.

6. Combine the tomato paste, herbs, water and garlic in a pan. Allow to simmer for 15 minutes.

7. Place half cup of tomato sauce in a baking dish.

8. Spread the chicken in a single layer then pour the tomato sauce and top with the mozzarella.

9. Bake for 10 minutes at 400 degrees. Serve warm.